Y0-ALD-284

LET'S LOOK AT BODY SYSTEMS!

RILEY'S REMARKABLE RESPIRATORY SYSTEM

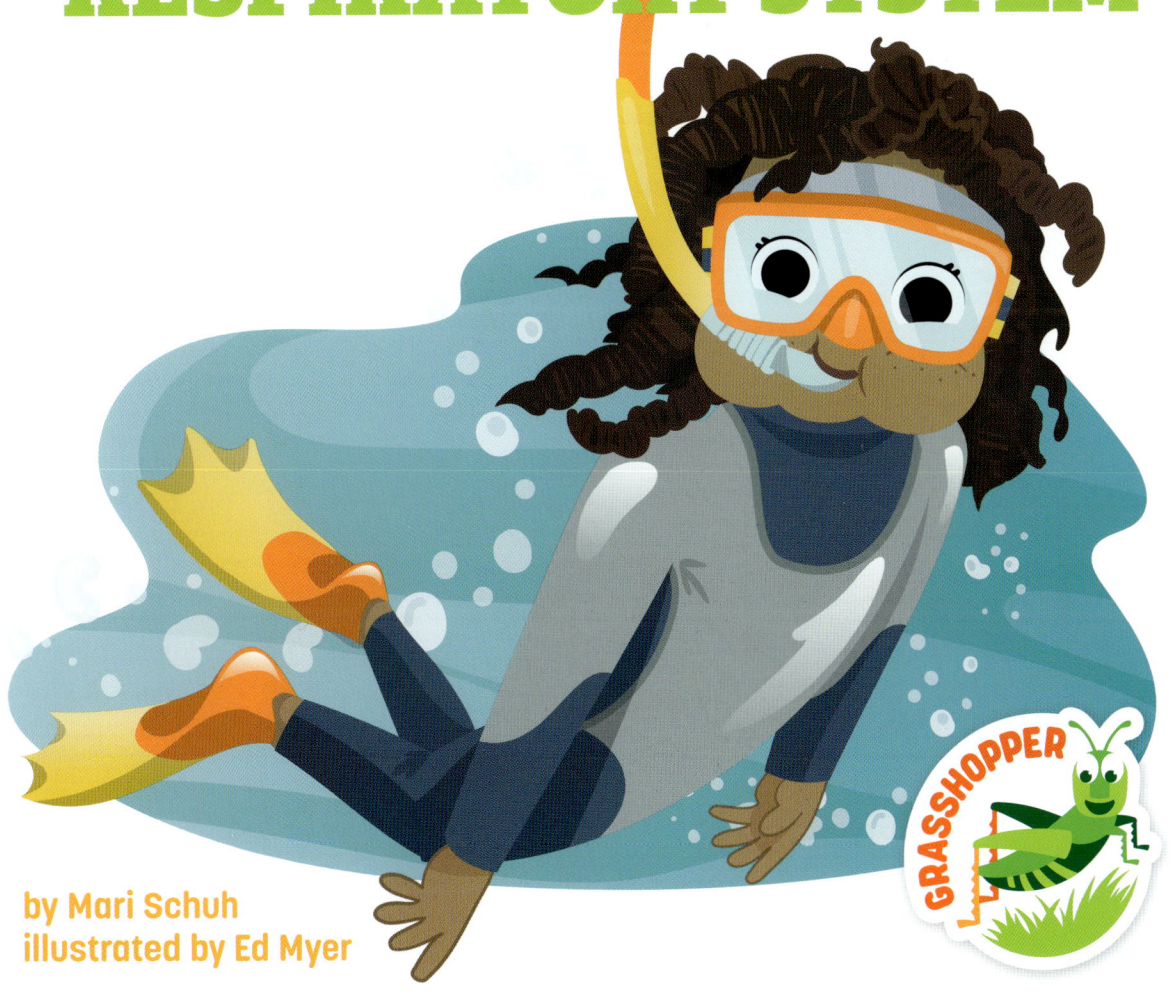

by Mari Schuh
illustrated by Ed Myer

GRASSHOPPER

Tools for Parents & Teachers

Grasshopper Books enhance imagination and introduce the earliest readers to fiction with fun storylines and illustrations. The easy-to-read text supports early reading experiences with repetitive sentence patterns and sight words.

Before Reading
- Discuss the cover illustration. What do they see?
- Look at the glossary together. Discuss the words.

Read the Book
- Read the book to the child, or have him or her read independently.
- "Walk" through the book and look at the illustrations. Who is the main character? What is happening in the story?

After Reading
- Prompt the child to think more. Ask: Think about a time when you were breathing hard and fast. What were you doing? How did your respiratory system help you?

Grasshopper Books are published by Jump!
5357 Penn Avenue South
Minneapolis, MN 55419
www.jumplibrary.com

Copyright © 2022 Jump! International copyright reserved in all countries. No part of this book may be reproduced in any form without written permission from the publisher.

Library of Congress Cataloging-in-Publication Data

Names: Schuh, Mari C., 1975- author. | Myer, Ed, illustrator.
Title: Riley's remarkable respiratory system / by Mari Schuh; illustrated by Ed Myer.
Description: Minneapolis, Minnesota: Jump!, Inc., [2022]
Series: Let's look at body systems! | Includes index.
Audience: Ages 7-10
Identifiers: LCCN 2021038063 (print)
LCCN 2021038064 (ebook)
ISBN 9781636906508 (hardcover)
ISBN 9781636906515 (paperback)
ISBN 9781636906522 (ebook)
Subjects: LCSH: Respiratory organs–Juvenile literature. Respiration–Juvenile literature. | Lungs–Juvenile literature.
Classification: LCC QP121 .S275 2022 (print)
LCC QP121 (ebook) | DDC 612.2–dc23
LC record available at https://lccn.loc.gov/2021038063
LC ebook record available at https://lccn.loc.gov/2021038064

Editor: Jenna Gleisner
Direction and Layout: Anna Peterson
Illustrator: Ed Myer

Printed in the United States of America at Corporate Graphics in North Mankato, Minnesota.

Table of Contents

Big Breaths	4
Let's Review!	22
Where in the Body?	23
To Learn More	23
Glossary	24
Index	24

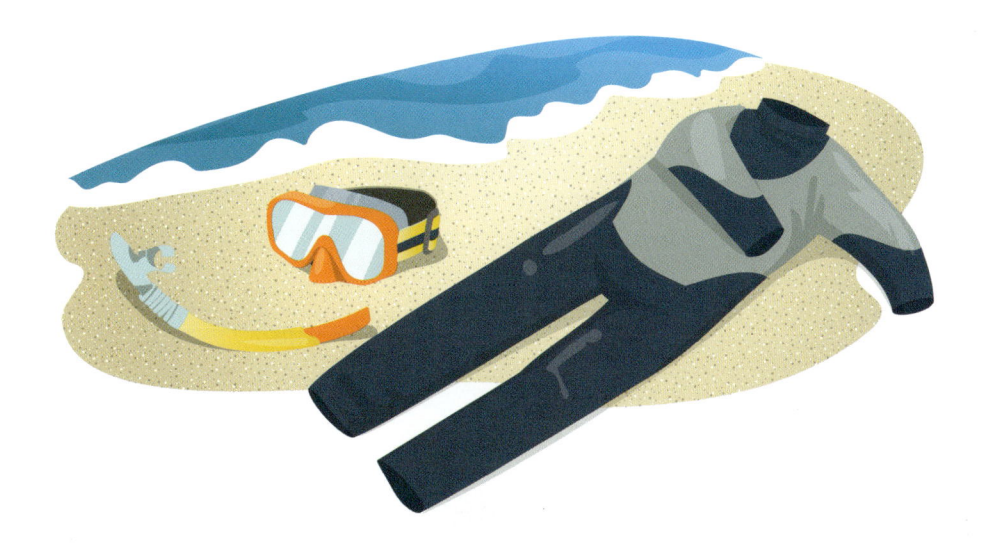

Big Breaths

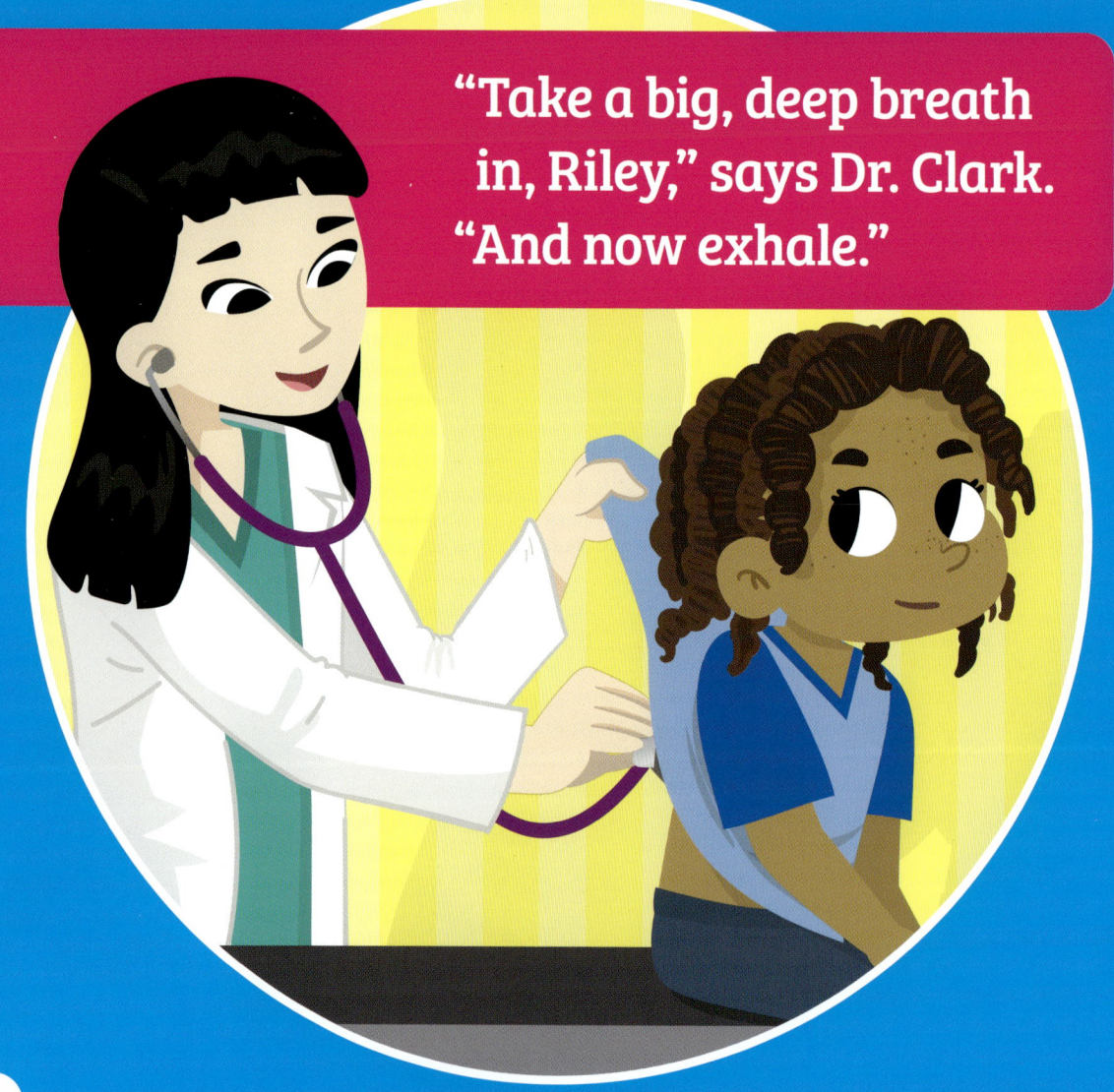

"Take a big, deep breath in, Riley," says Dr. Clark. "And now exhale."

"Your lungs sound great!" Dr. Clark says.

"What do my lungs do, anyway?" asks Riley.

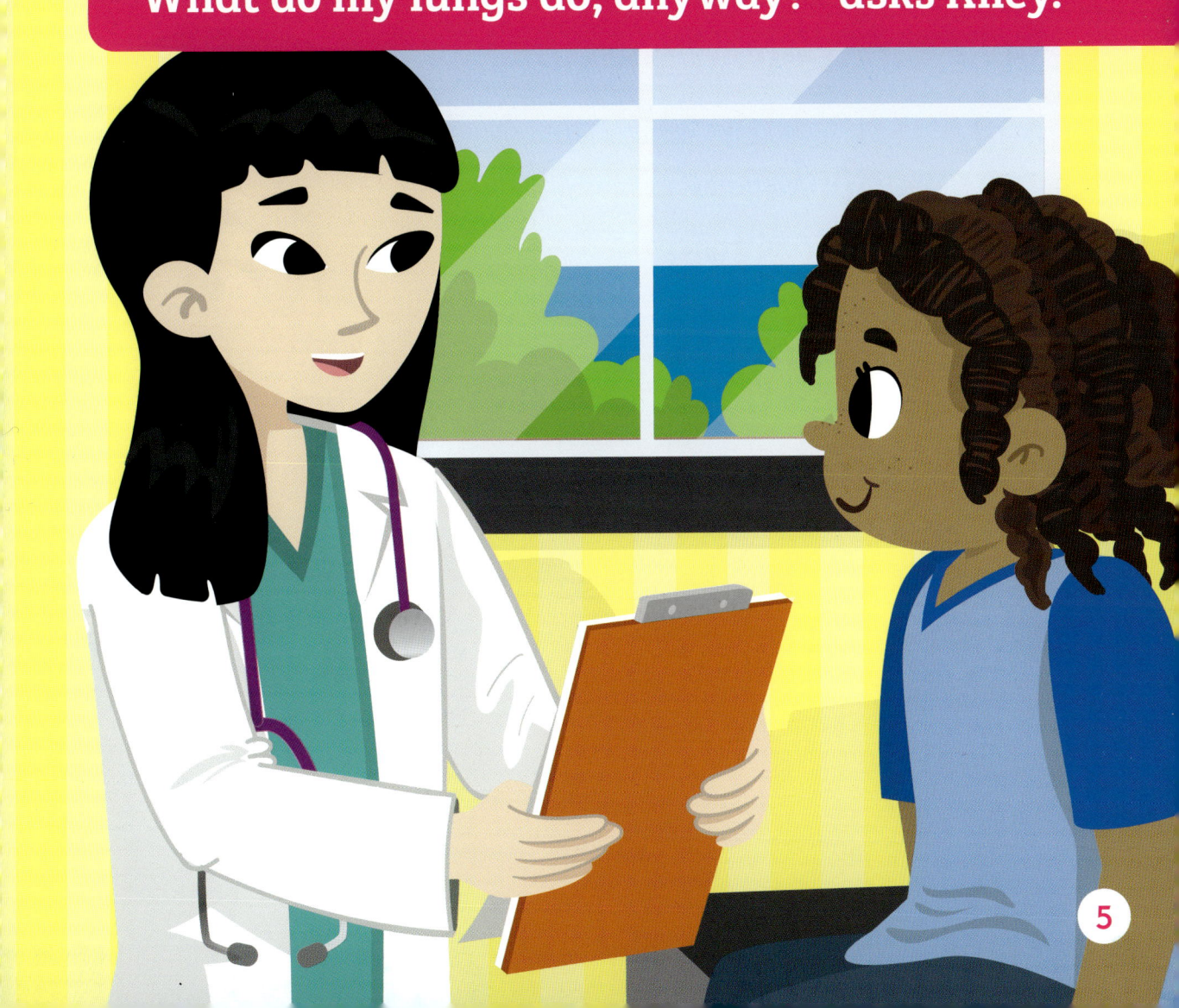

"Lungs help us breathe air. Oxygen in the air keeps us alive. Lungs also get rid of waste, like carbon dioxide. They are an important part of your respiratory system. Take a look!" Dr. Clark says.

"Air goes in your nose or mouth. It travels down your trachea. Then it goes through tubes called bronchi, which go into your lungs."

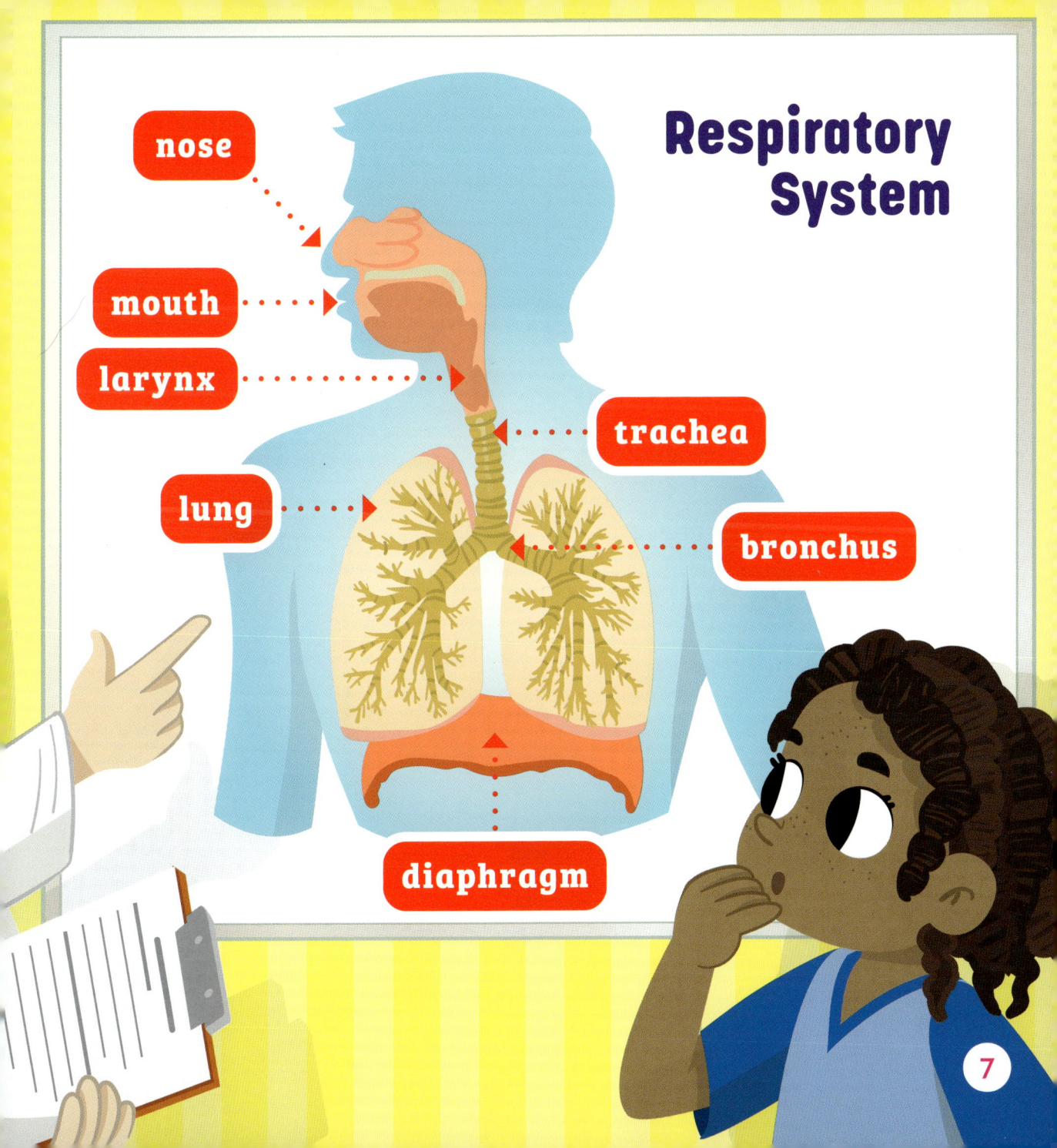

Respiratory System

- nose
- mouth
- larynx
- trachea
- lung
- bronchus
- diaphragm

"How is there room in there?" asks Riley.

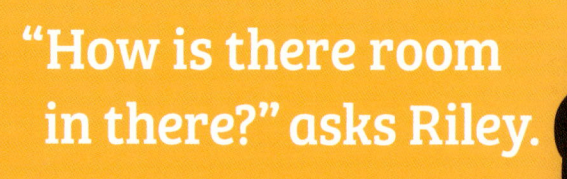

"Take a deep breath in," says Dr. Clark. "Do you feel your chest expand? Your diaphragm moves down so your lungs can fill with air."

diaphragm

"When you exhale, your diaphragm moves up and your chest goes back to its normal size," Dr. Clark says.

"That seems pretty simple!" says Riley.

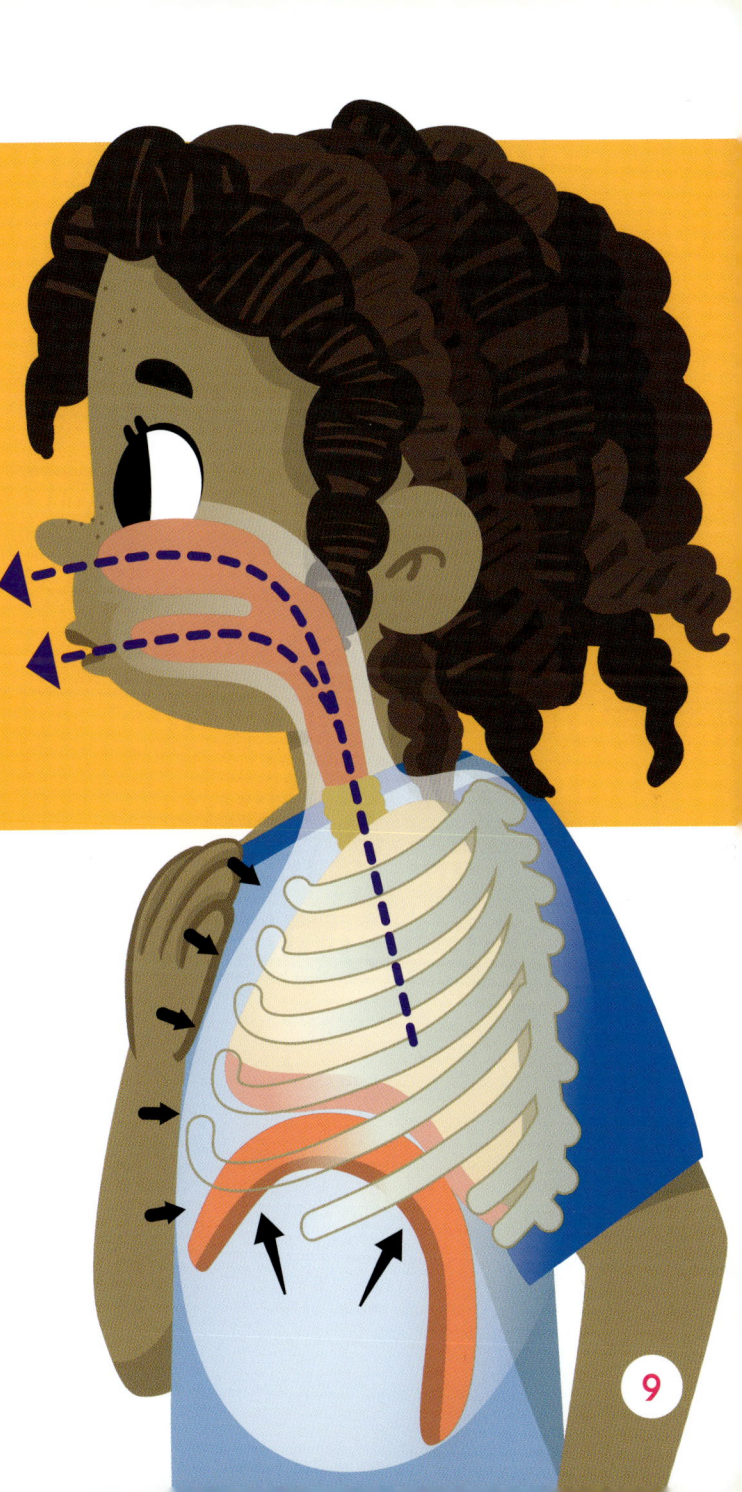

"Actually, your respiratory system is pretty remarkable," says Dr. Clark. "Many parts work together."

"The bronchi branch out into smaller tubes called bronchioles. They end in tiny air sacs called alveoli. Your lungs have more than 600 million alveoli!"

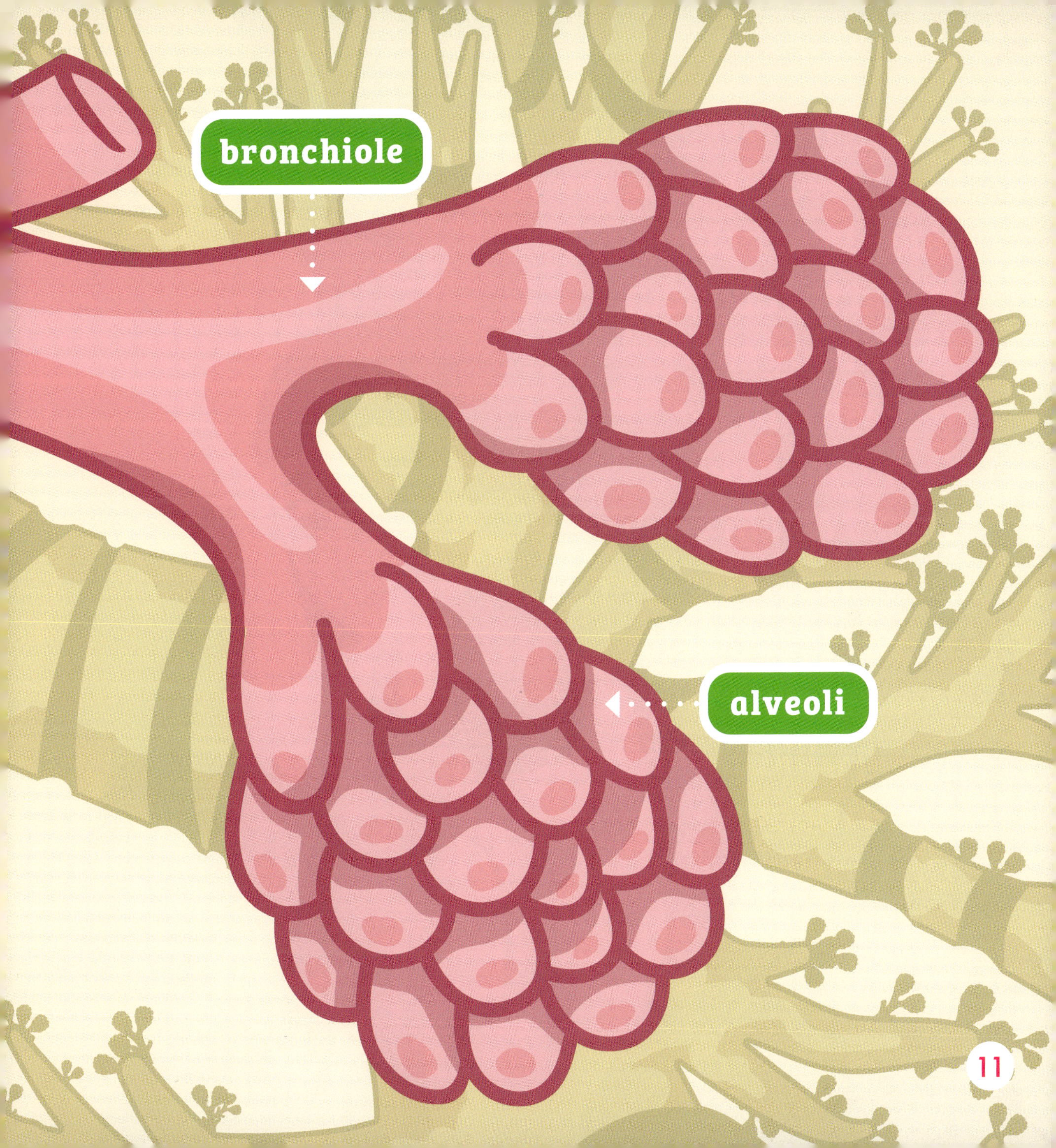
bronchiole
alveoli

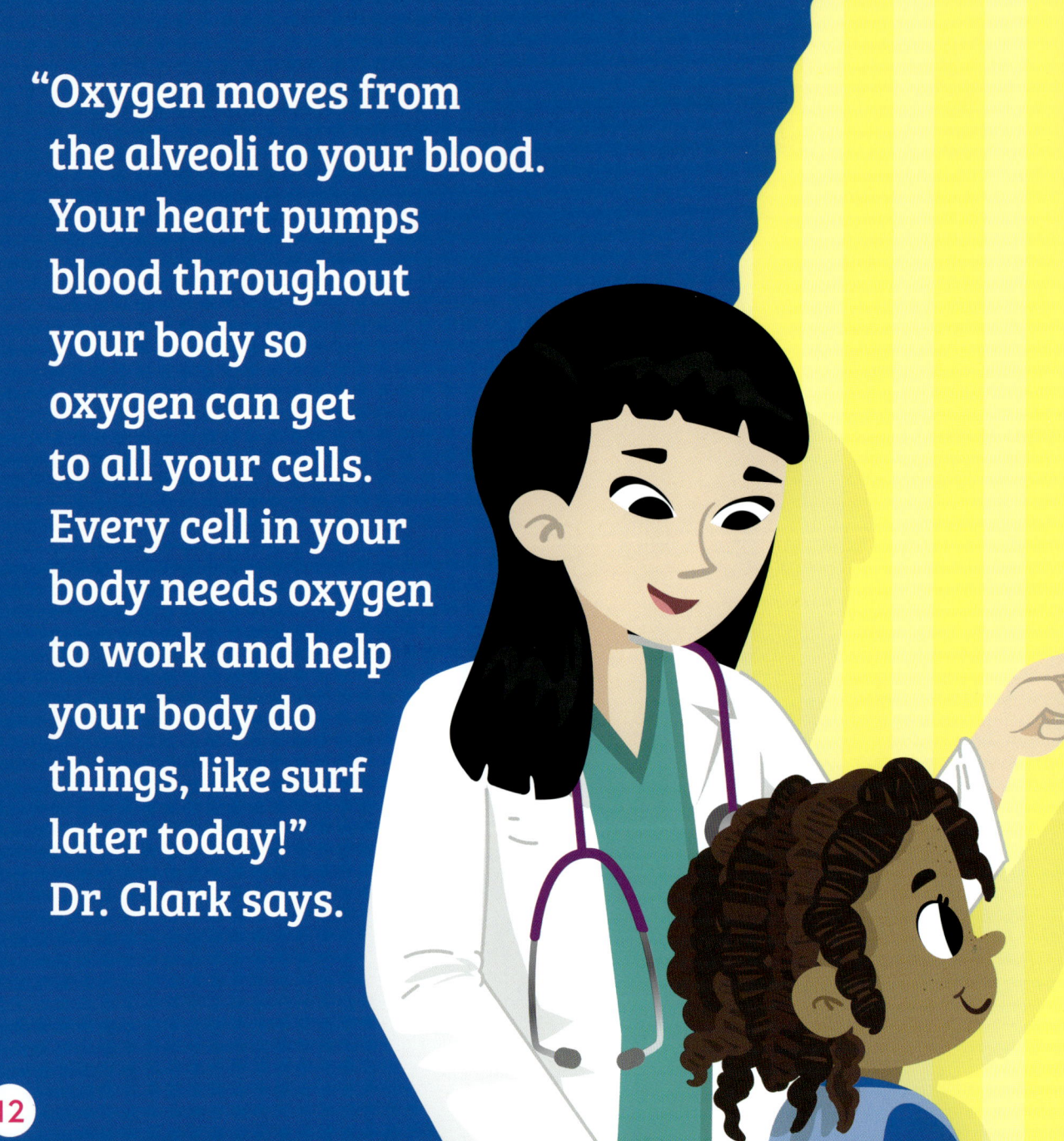

"Oxygen moves from the alveoli to your blood. Your heart pumps blood throughout your body so oxygen can get to all your cells. Every cell in your body needs oxygen to work and help your body do things, like surf later today!" Dr. Clark says.

heart

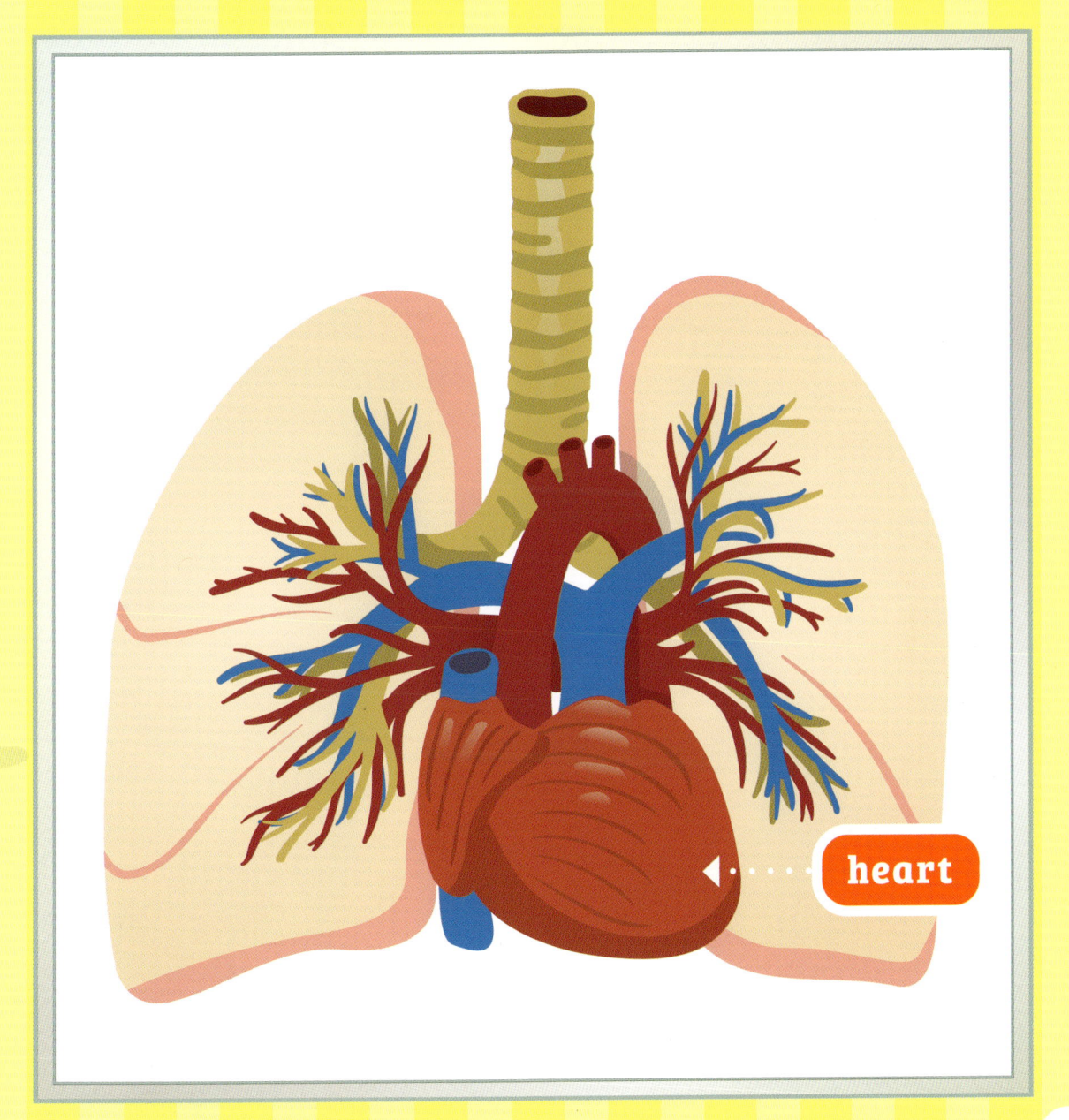

"I can feel my lungs working!" Riley says later as she and her dad paddle their surfboards.

"That's right!" Riley's dad says. "Do you notice that you breathe faster, too? That's because your body needs more oxygen to work harder."

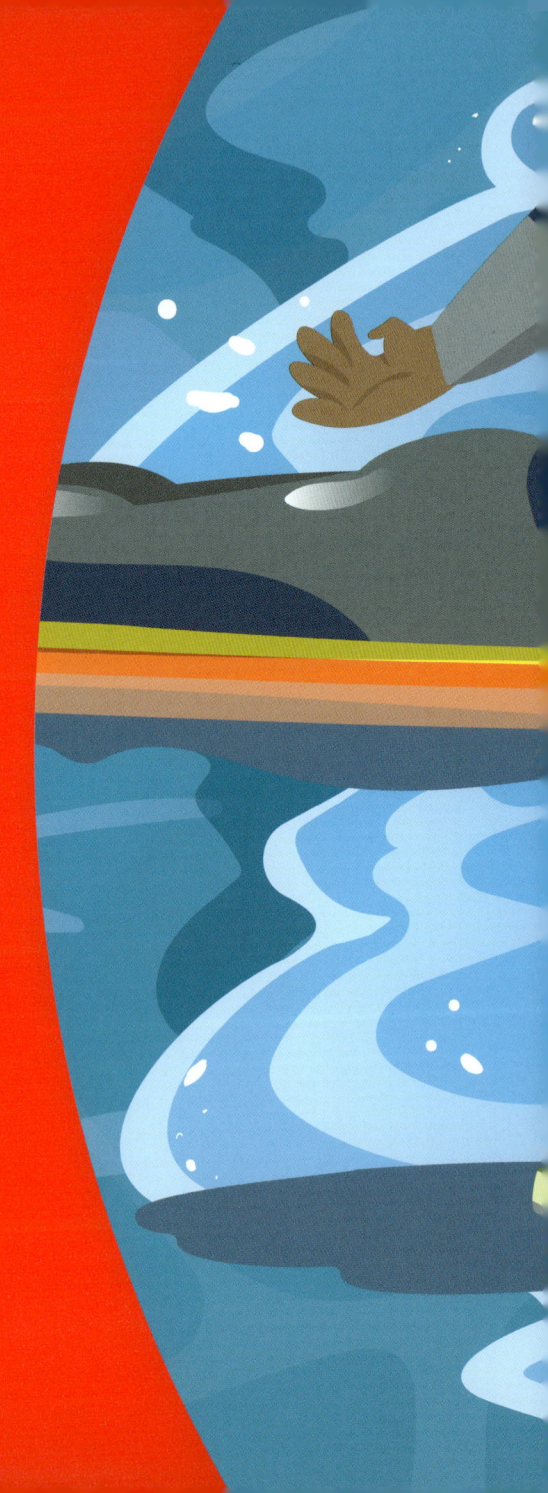

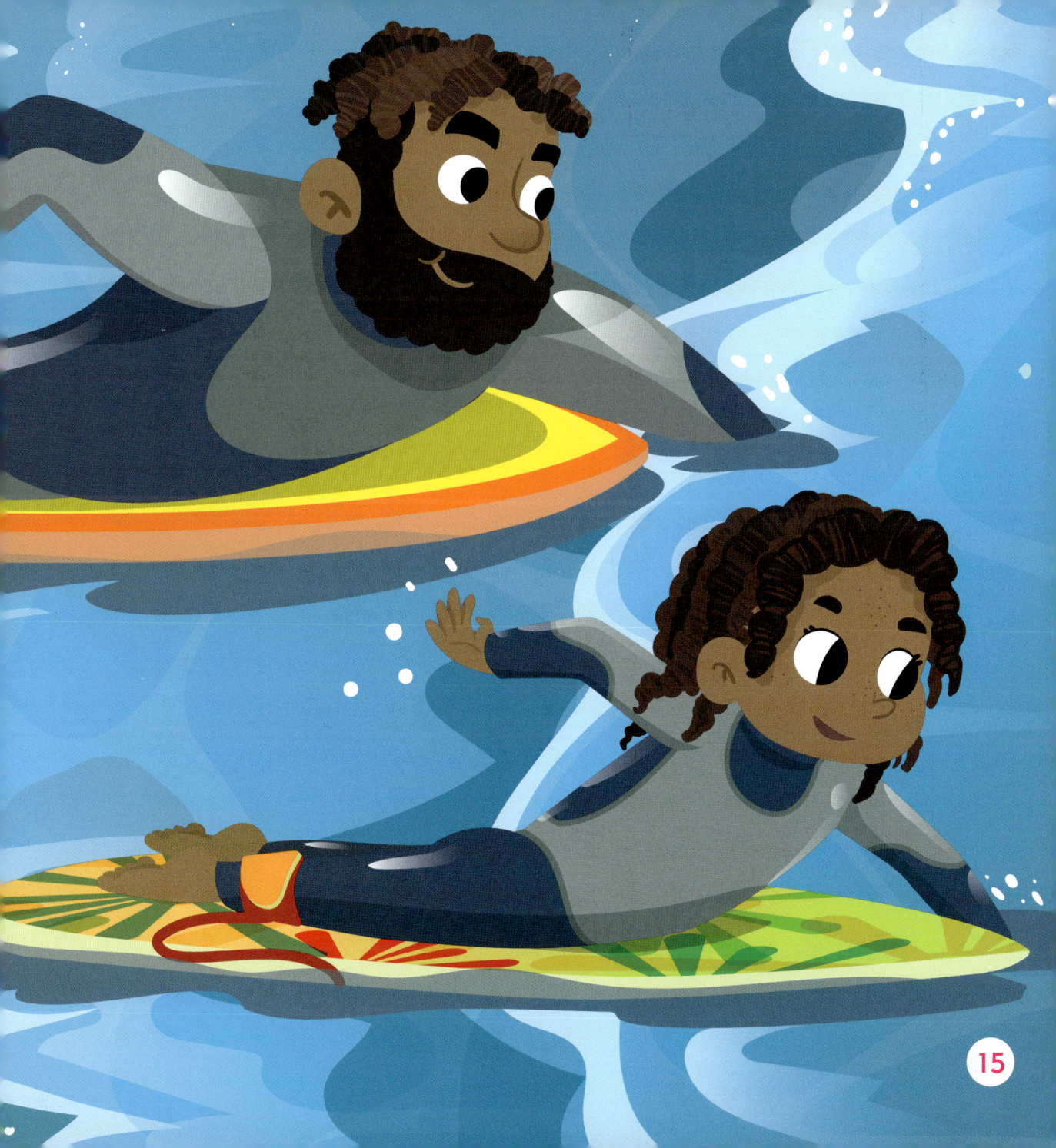

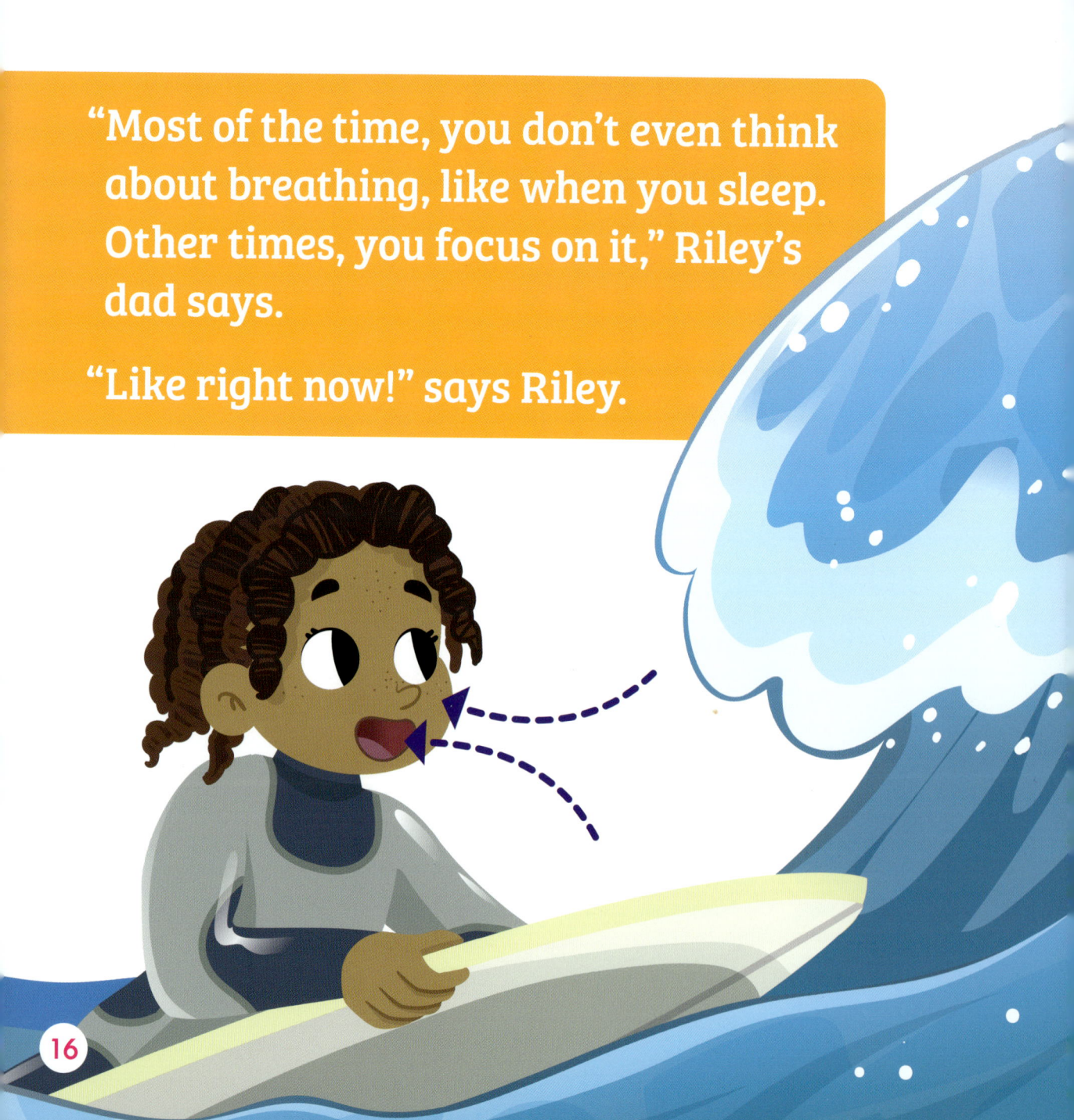

"Most of the time, you don't even think about breathing, like when you sleep. Other times, you focus on it," Riley's dad says.

"Like right now!" says Riley.

Riley holds her breath as she swims under a wave.

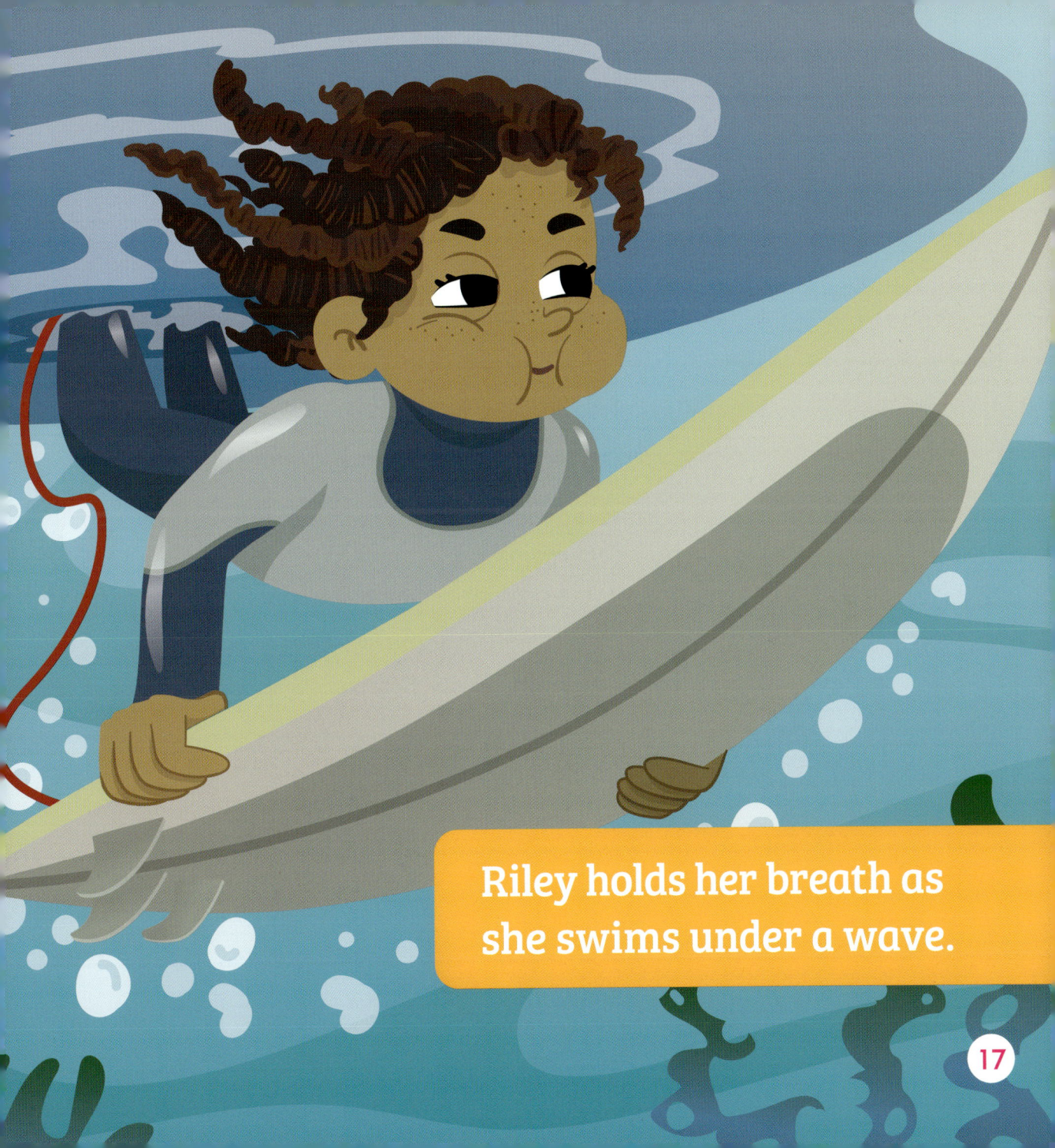

"Nice job, Riley!" says her dad.

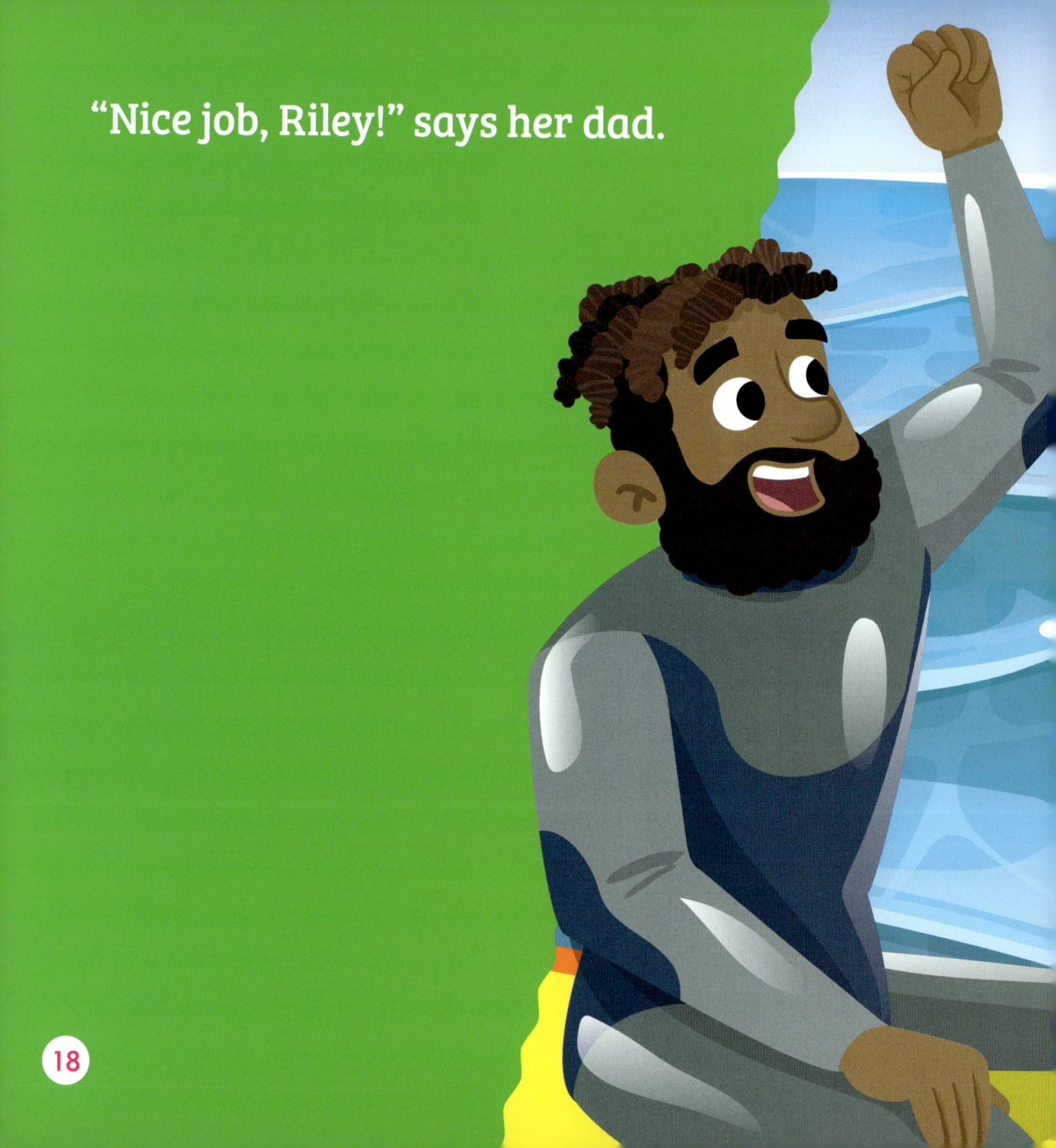

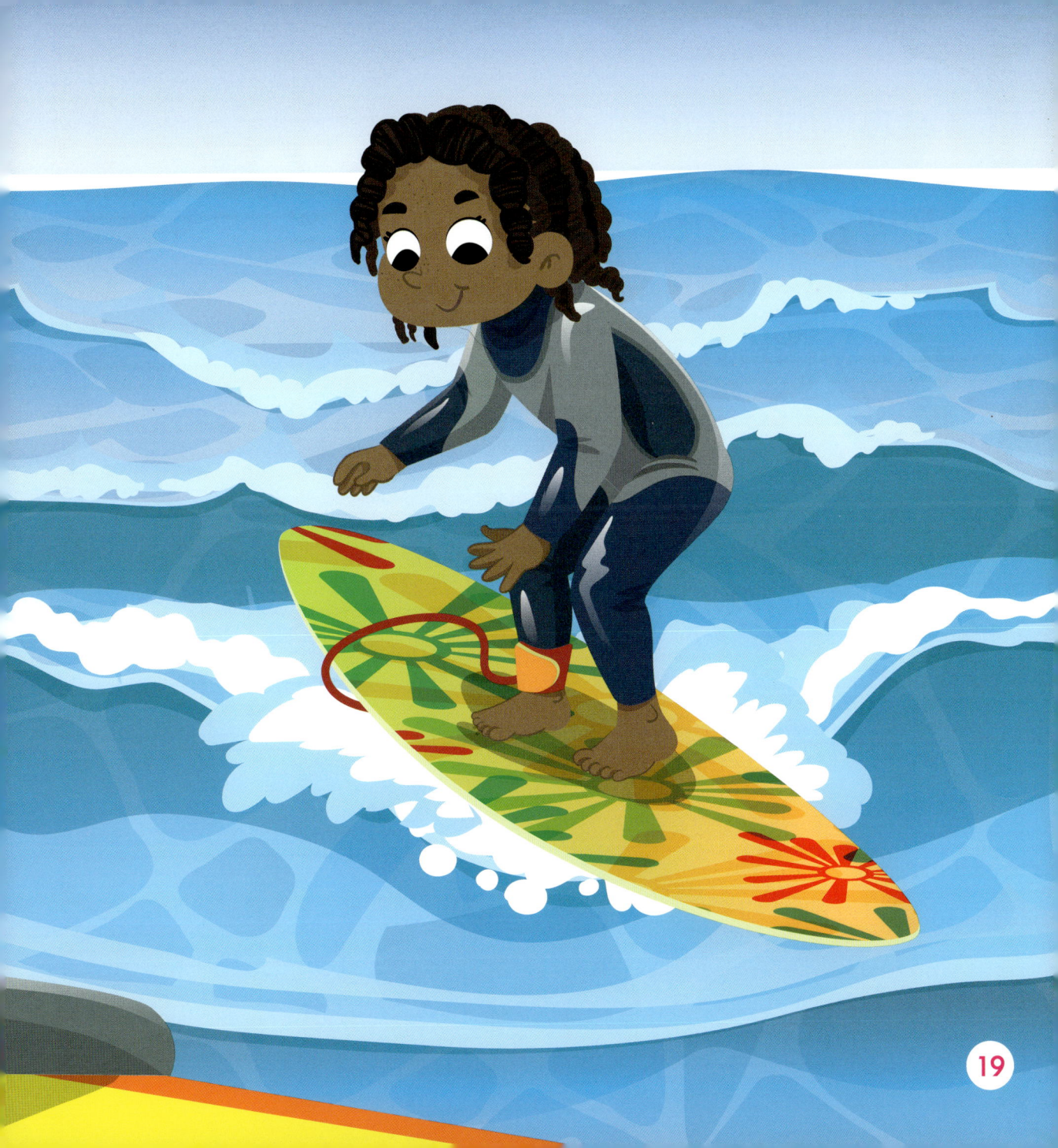

"Swimming and surfing make our lungs stronger," Riley's dad says. "So does eating healthy foods and washing our hands to keep germs away."

"I do all of that," says Riley. "That's why I can take big breaths and catch BIG waves!"

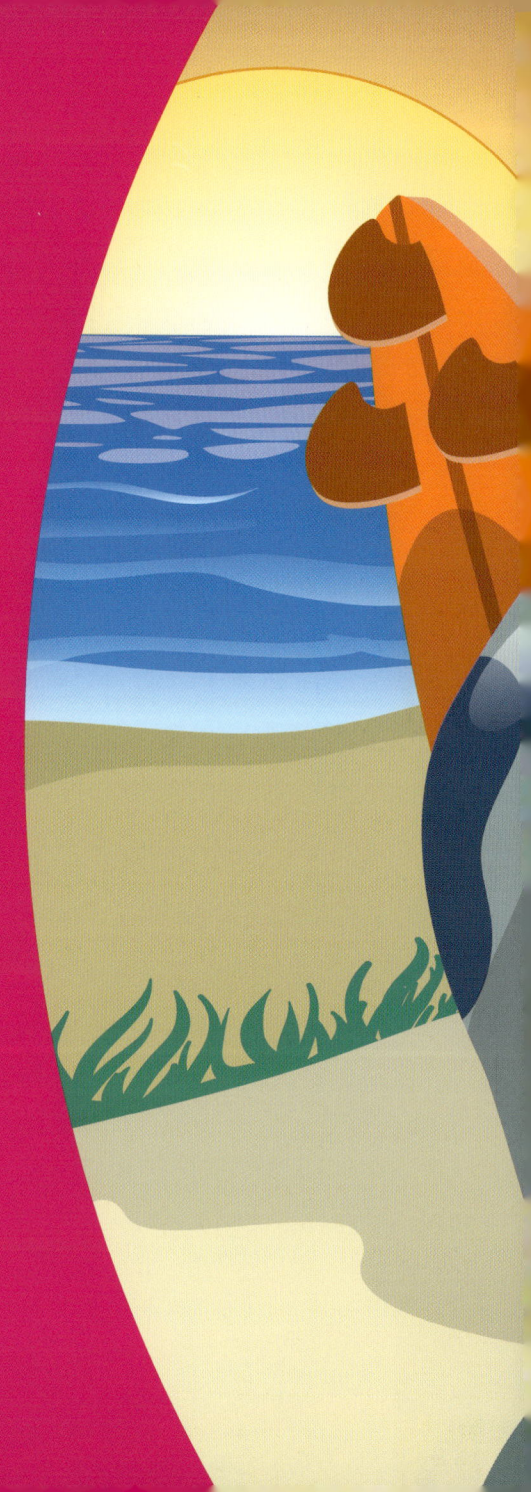

21

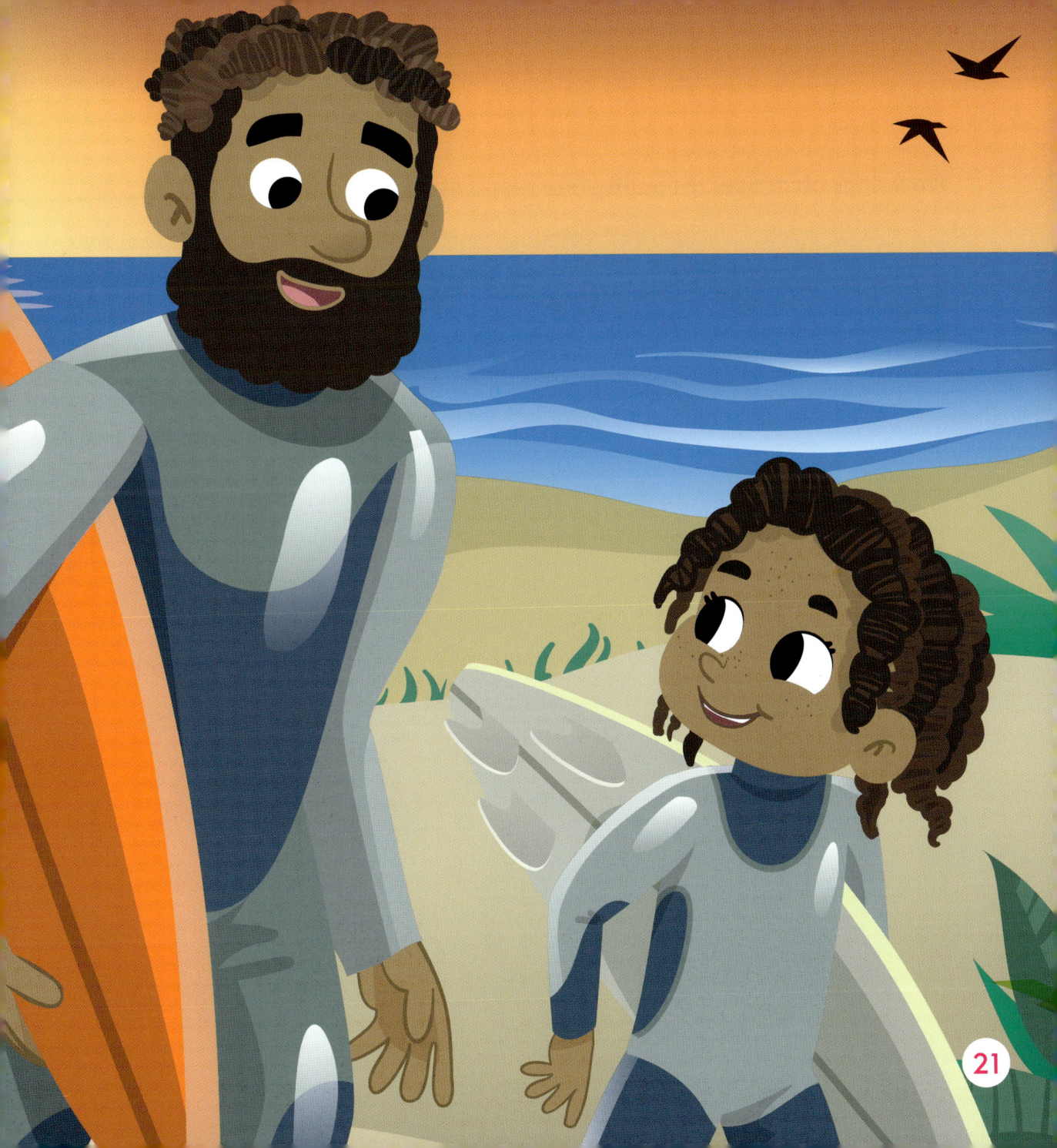

Let's Review!

How does air travel through your respiratory system? Let's take a look!

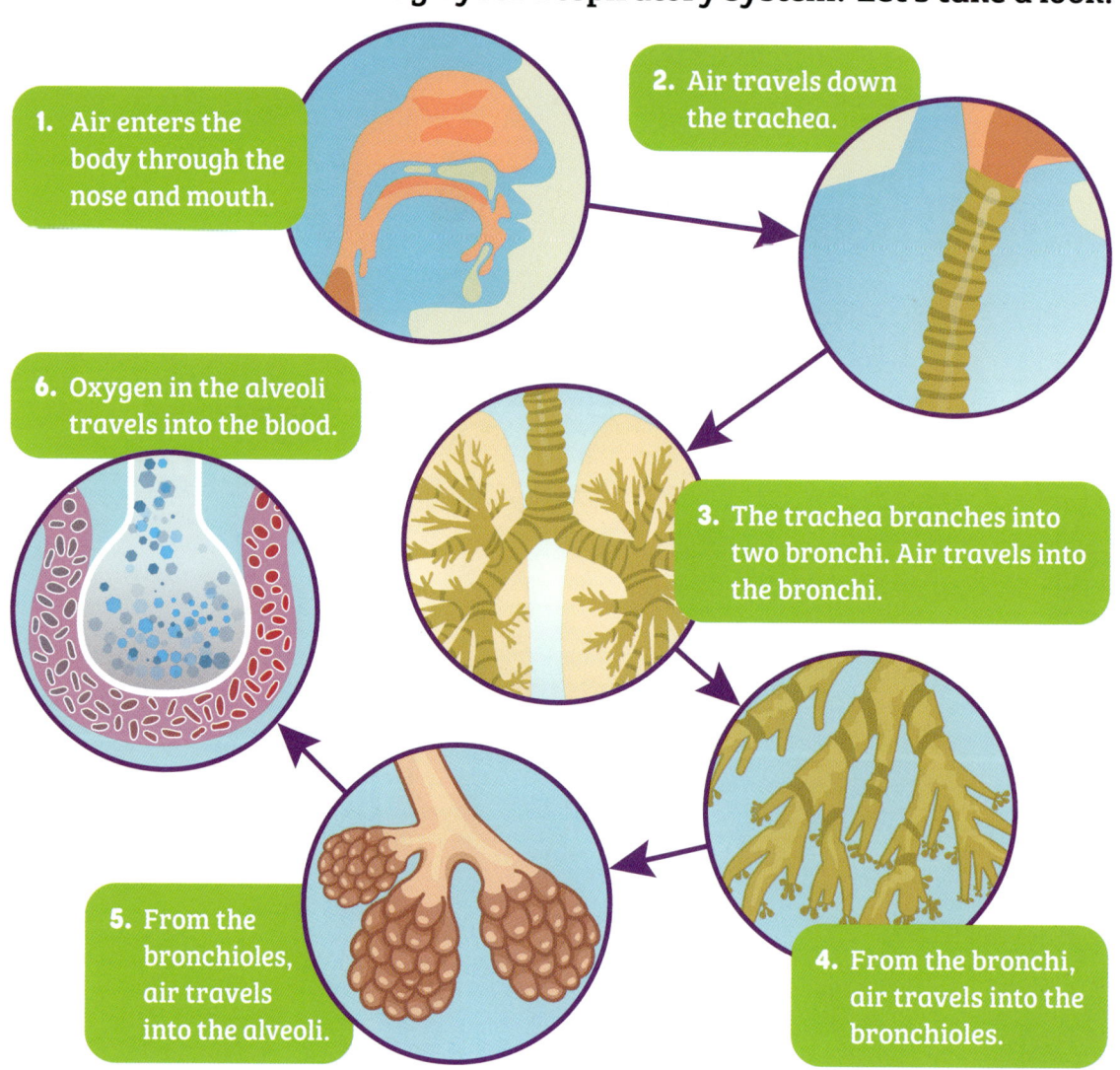

1. Air enters the body through the nose and mouth.

2. Air travels down the trachea.

3. The trachea branches into two bronchi. Air travels into the bronchi.

4. From the bronchi, air travels into the bronchioles.

5. From the bronchioles, air travels into the alveoli.

6. Oxygen in the alveoli travels into the blood.

Where in the Body?

Here are the major parts of the respiratory system.

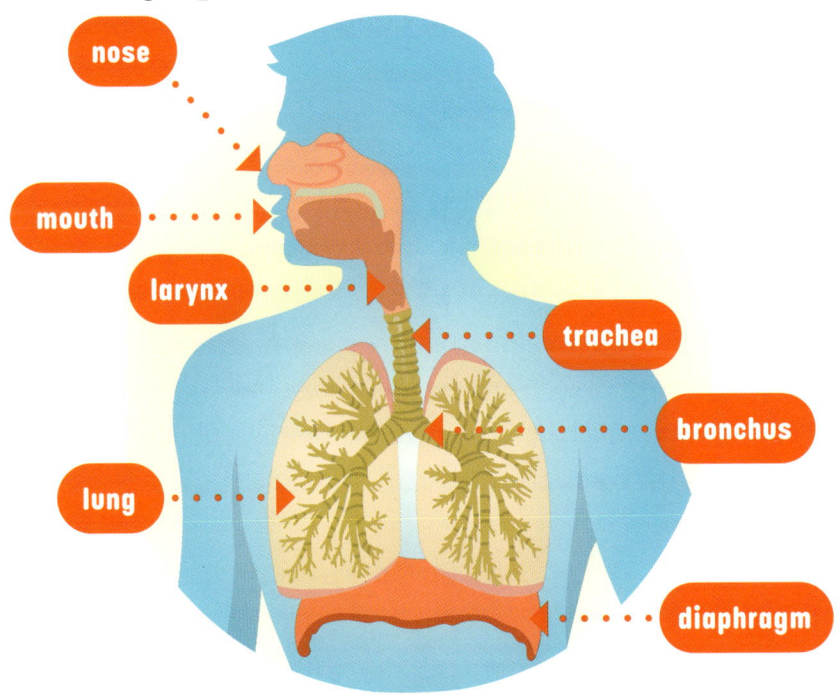

- nose
- mouth
- larynx
- trachea
- bronchus
- lung
- diaphragm

To Learn More

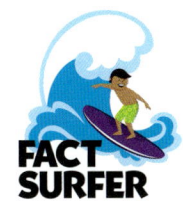

Finding more information is as easy as 1, 2, 3.

1. Go to www.factsurfer.com
2. Enter "**Riley'sremarkablerespiratorysystem**" into the search box.
3. Choose your book to see a list of websites.

23

Glossary

alveoli: Tiny air sacs at the end of the bronchioles in the lungs.

bronchi: The two main tubes that branch off the trachea.

bronchioles: Small tubes that branch off the bronchi.

carbon dioxide: A gas that humans and animals breathe out.

cells: The smallest parts of living things. A microscope is needed to see cells.

diaphragm: The wall of muscle in your lower chest that separates the lungs from the stomach area and assists in breathing.

expand: To become larger.

lungs: The two baglike organs inside your chest that fill with air when you breathe. The lungs supply the blood with oxygen and rid the blood of carbon dioxide.

oxygen: A gas found in the air, which humans need to breathe and live.

trachea: The main trunk of the respiratory system. Also called the windpipe.

Index

air 6, 8, 10
alveoli 10, 12
blood 12
breath 4, 8, 17, 20
breathe 6, 14, 16
bronchi 6, 10
bronchioles 10
carbon dioxide 6
chest 8, 9

diaphragm 8, 9
heart 12
lungs 5, 6, 8, 10, 14, 20
mouth 6
nose 6
oxygen 6, 12, 14
surf 12, 20
swims 17, 20
trachea 6